Refusing The Needle

A Diabetic's Natural Journey To Kick-Ass Health

Russell Stamets

Every human being is the author of his own health or disease.
~ Buddha

Table of Contents

WHY READ THIS BOOK

Have Diabetes? Tired of hearing people say "that's terrible"? And agreeing with them? Disgusted with the only option offered—the rest of your life as a lab rat, with devices, needles, and 24/7 monitoring? If it's yes to any of those questions, read on.

I was just a regular 49 year old beer-guzzling, french fry lovin' guy, in seemingly great health when told I had diabetes. And not just the common Type 2 that millions are getting-- my doc suspected that I had a Type 1 variety called Latent Autoimmune Diabetes in Adults (LADA). Hearing the *autoimmune* part of that was a punch in the stomach. Type 2's have a fantastic chance of controlling their high blood sugar with pills and curing it with diet. But the Type 1 autoimmune varieties are advised that the attack on their pancreas is irreversible. We're told, "You'll need a daily shot of insulin forever". Irreversible? Forever? Talk about a "just shoot me now" moment.

That moment was almost 3 years ago. Miraculously, I've never required insulin injections. My blood sugar levels are normal. I figured out a way to heal my body with diet, a few supplements, exercise, yoga, acupuncture, and meditation… I know. Go ahead and roll your eyes. *I'm just sayin'!*

Let me tell you what I did, and why. Make up your own mind. Form your own plan. The thing you might find hardest to believe is that I count my diabetes as a benefit. Because without it, if you're like me, you wouldn't get off your butt to do something. OK, so maybe you are actually sitting on your butt while reading this, but bear with me. The point is that *your new body and mind will be as great a result as curing diabetes.*

I had one lucky break. My doc has a passion for evidence-based medicine. He said I could buy time if I wanted to try to find another approach. He warned that in his opinion, the road ended in insulin no matter what, but that starting insulin immediately had no better outcome than waiting until it was required. That gift of time was critical. He said any endocrinologist he knew would probably disapprove of the delay and would order insulin immediately. Based on the general disbelief I encounter from anyone in the *Diabetes Establishment* regarding my story, my doc appears to be a rare, open minded member of his profession.

I vowed to wisely use the time he gave me.

My first instinct told me that if western medicine was a dead end, why not look east? I went to a good RN friend who runs a world-renowned Integrated Therapies department of the local hospital. I'd never used any of her services, but I knew her staff offered all kinds of massage, acupuncture, and more. If anyone could give me a trustworthy opinion of the potential for eastern options, Michelle could. She introduced me to Jane who is both an acupuncturist and practicing Chinese herbalist. In addition to weekly acupuncture, which at the very least is critical for managing the all-important stress driver, I've leaned heavily on Jane's nutrition and supplement expertise. The very first recommendation Jane gave when we met in February, 2011, was to quit all alcohol. I'd already ditched the rum and beer and had switched to a couple of glasses of red wine. Even my doc thought that was reasonable. But Jane said any stress on the liver equals stress on the pancreas. That was a pivotal moment in trust and commitment. I went all in for this hand. The bottle of merlot I'd bought the day before is still in the cupboard, unopened. Too bad it's not the good stuff which will get better with age.

I used a news reader on my android phone to scan daily for bits of science drowned in the fire hose of information hitting us these days. I was looking for studies specific to blood sugar management, long-term damage control, and finding a root cure. I would forward them to Jane for her opinion, and if it was about a supplement to try, to get her recommendation for dosage. It appears now that spring 2011 was a good period of time to be researching diabetes/autoimmune science. For several months there was a steady stream of clues to follow up. By May my regimen was pretty set. Nothing since has shown up to prompt any modifications. My own daily tracking provided other clues. The role of animal saturated fat is an example of something that barely appears in the science.

I could cut stuff out one at a time to test and see what really worked to lower my A1c so much, but I hate to do it. Everything I'm doing is either harmless or proven to be good for you aside from any diabetes-related benefit.

A common musing of mine, which I'm sure people around me get tired of hearing, is that people don't die from diabetes. They die from *complications* (hate that word). The complications, including cardiovascular, kidney, and neurodegenerative, are the same things that the majority of non-diabetics die from. Diabetics just die from them sooner and have a few other fun likelihoods, like retinopathy. The connections are not serendipitous. Many of these chronic conditions are inflammatory or autoimmune related and share similar causes like genetics or toxic diet. And anything found to reduce inflammation, help the immune system, or mitigate long term cell damage likewise synergistically helps with this whole range of ills, including diabetes.

If I haven't already put you to sleep or scared you off, the plan for the rest of this book is to give you more detail on what I've done, and why. In addition to my take on the science, or lack of, and some of the apparent market motivations for how diabetes is treated, I'm going to try to give you a peek inside my head. Successfully winning the mental game may be the biggest part of the solution I've found. Even though everyone's starting place and game board will be a little different, the goal is the same. And so are many of the obstacles to beating diabetes. The manner in which I stumbled over them to get here will help you chart your course.

The least controversial part of my message is that even folks that aren't sick will be happier, healthier, and live longer by following my plan. More accepted, but certainly bucking the financial interest headwind is my suggestion that Type 2 diabetics and other chronic disease sufferers can cure themselves by diet and lifestyle changes alone.

Reversal of an autoimmune disease (Type 1 LADA Diabetes) is the most controversial part of my story. As I warn that insulin may be overprescribed, or too quickly ordered, the establishment is moving the other direction. Voices advocating that more Type 2 diabetics should start insulin, and that Type 1 LADA's should start sooner, are loud. The money trail behind these voices is troubling. It often leads to Big Pharma and the multi-billion dollar insulin and device industry. There's a growing body of evidence for alternative treatments, but they're generally not patentable, and therefore not of interest to corporate sources of research funding or corporate owned media. LADA, in particular, is barely studied because no one will spend the money for large-scale trials that need to go for 12 years.

Perhaps it would make more sense to speak exclusively to the diabetes population. Several hundred million is a sizeable audience to focus on. Type 1 and 2 diabetics are theoretically more motivated to hear about a *cure*. They have more obviously immediate benefit (like not dying young or losing a limb). I'm showing diabetics a stark choice between a punctured, tethered, fretful life and one that's an upgrade from the pre-diabetes self.

But on the quality of life scale, you have the typical diabetic at the low end, a regular, healthy, normal person up a few ticks to the right, and then this upgraded body I'm touting, far up out of sight on the *wouldn't-have-dreamed-possible* side. I'm finding it extremely difficult not to attempt to communicate this discovery to normal, non-diabetics too. It's a much harder sell. As I've stated before, I thought I was Superman before diabetes. I was strong, healthy, felt great. I would have scoffed if told that what I thought was strong, healthy, and feeling great was a long way from the best possible. Sounds obvious, but it's a fact that if your life's not in immediate danger, the priority rating is pretty low for experimenting with clean living. For normal folks there are so many days from now until death that the craved caramel latte right now seems insignificant as a harmful contribution. Tomorrow is soon enough to start. And how could giving up these little sins-that-make-life-bearable outweigh some dubious gain in wellness?

If you decide this approach is right for you, some people will think you are crazy. Most of the critics are well meaning. I'm sure most endocrinologists believe they've read the evidence (and lack of) in an un-biased way. And the tens of thousands of current insulin-using diabetics are sincere when they adamantly insist you're far better off (and in fact will only survive) shooting insulin. There's nothing to be gained by reminding them that they have had to rationalize the extreme hit to their lifestyle that it represents. Think about it. If a natural, simple, more effective way to control their blood sugar existed, and they chose a 24/7/365/lifetime finger-pricking nightmare instead… how could they live with themselves? But of course, they didn't *choose* it. They were told there is *no* option. Just like you've been told, or will be, and just like I was told. But if you're reading this, maybe you'll see the choice.

Are you ready to take charge of your own health? If that's a "yes", read on and I'll give you the information and tools to make your own choices. No crossed fingers though. If you take this road to Shangri-La, you'll only make it over the pass with honest commitment. You'll actually have to prove you love your life enough to change it and *leave your victim behind.*

WHAT IS DIABETES

For those not already experts on the flavors of diabetes, let me provide a quick primer. Type 1 and Type 2 are really two different diseases at both ends of a spectrum that has combination varieties in between. They both result in abnormally high levels of blood glucose. High BG (also called blood sugar) causes lots of problems that can kill you either sooner or later. There are 2 ways those levels can get high and that pretty much defines the difference between Type 1 and 2. Your pancreas creates the insulin that allows your body to use the glucose for fuel. This action happens in cells that can become resistant to insulin. A Type 1 has a pancreas that's not producing enough insulin. A Type 2 has cells that are resistant to insulin. Either way blood sugar (glucose) goes up.

Type 2 is far more common. It can be acquired through unhealthy lifestyle. And it can be controlled with medications or often reversed by discontinuing the eating of *crap*. Type 1 is genetic. It's an autoimmune disease that has the body attacking its own pancreas, killing the production of insulin. It's universally believed to be irreversible. People with Type 1 inject insulin constantly to prevent deadly blood glucose levels. The majority of Type 1's are diagnosed as kids, who at a certain age quickly lose their capacity to produce insulin. Currently, they have no option except injecting insulin for the rest of their lives. A recent development is the emergence of a variation of Type 1 that affects adults over 35. It's thought to be genetic and possibly triggered by stress and lousy diet. This variation is called Latent (or Late-onset) Autoimmune Diabetes in Adults. LADA takes longer to kill the pancreas than the juvenile version of Type 1. It can be 2-12 years between onset and when the insulin producing beta cells of the pancreas are so far gone that shots of insulin (or a pump) are necessary. Diet, exercise, medications, and everything that works for a Type 2 will work for a while with LADA, but with diminishing returns.

There are many variations from Type1 to the LADA varieties all the way to Type 2. This is why you will find so many different stories that might seem conflicting. Some Type 2's now appear to have a genetic component and some Type 1's still have some percentage of pancreas function. None of the traditional black and white statements are completely accurate. This is one of the main reasons you'll have to ask questions and figure out for yourself where your pin goes on the map, and where you should focus your efforts.

If you want more of the science, head online and you'll find out pretty quickly that the pancreas is pretty underrated. It's an ugly, hidden away organ, but complex, judged partly by what scientists still don't know about it. By comparison, the heart, which gets all the press, is just a pump. But the pancreas is an entire, multi-function chemistry lab. They still don't understand how it works normally, much less how the body's immune system malfunctions and decides to attack it. Sometimes, while reading the research, I wish I were a video game developer. Some of the narrative has promise:

***~ ~ ~ ***

On the oft-forgotten Pancreatic Continent you will find the Islets of Langerhans. And thereupon reside the talented Betacellites who labor tirelessly to produce the life sustaining Insulin, which they freely distribute to the rest of Bodyworld. Unfortunately, the planetary defender, Otto Imyoon, has cracked under the toxic stress of what the Russellverse rained down on him for several decades. He's delusionally shooting anything that moves, and the poor little Betas in particular are undergoing genocide. Otto orders his imperial storm troopers, the TH1, to launch daily sorties, wreaking havoc across the Islets. The planetary legislature has dispatched scores of TH2 envoys, but reports of their efforts range from ineffectual to complicit. And then there's the shadowy world of the Kevorkian RNAgents, enticing the Betas to suicide. Will the toxic flood stop? Will Otto Imyoon regain his senses? Can the Betas rebuild? Will they want to? Stay tuned!

WHO SAYS IMPOSSIBLE

The reason western medicine writes off your pancreas as soon as antibodies are found in your blood (showing your body is attacking it) is because they don't have a clue how to stop it. It's why insulin, a 100 year old treatment that clumsily attempts to address one symptom (not even the cause) is all a newly diagnosed Type 1 diabetic will be offered.

Cancer is often called the *plague* of our times, but the title should really be awarded to *Autoimmune Disorders*. Cancer is just one of more than 80 that that are autoimmune related. Besides cancer and Type 1 diabetes, Celiac Disease, Rheumatoid Arthritis, Multiple Sclerosis, Addison's, Lupus, Graves, and even eczema fall within its path of destruction. This is one reason that even Type 2 diabetics, whose diabetes is not directly autoimmune related might still want to stay tuned in here. Even if you're currently healthy, what are the odds that you or someone you know will have one or more of this lengthy list of common conditions? Western medicine is working round the clock to find answers, but it may take a while. And that's assuming they're looking in the right direction. Reading the studies, there appear to be thousands of chemical reactions associated with all the proteins and cell types identified with specific immune system responses. Legions of mice are giving their lives for each miniscule jigsaw piece. But are we looking too closely? Maybe instead of trying to monkey wrench the body machine with tools we don't even have, we should step back and consider simpler things like the fuel we dump in it. The only workable answer may be in the *fringe* evidence like mine and others', suggesting that a healthy diet can stop the short circuit in the immune system. As the stories of cancer survivors and reversed Type 1 diabetes cases (like me) continue to proliferate, the idea that eliminating processed foods and radically reducing stress can cure autoimmune disorders may become more mainstream. But don't hold your breath. As my conspiracy-theory side will periodically remind, you can't patent local fresh vegetables and meditation, so who is going to spend money to research it or report on it?

~~~

I am Anecdotal
the tangled web of variables I weave
gives shivers to the evidence-based
supplements, diet, meditation, oh my!
which one prodded this pancreas to produce again?
I could say I'm sorry to not have spent the years required
to have double-blind tested
each and every part of my solution...
but I'm not

~~~

So be prepared. You may have to listen to someone who paid an awful lot for a great medical degree tell you that what you want to do (what I've done) is impossible. If that happens, you can always find a doctor with a more open mind. My doc didn't think much of what I tried would work, but he respected my desire to try, and his reading of the evidence was that I had time to try to buy time.

A couple of recent reports have been published refuting the idea that a Type 1 diabetic's pancreas is dead. The first, by Professor Bart Roep of Leiden University Medical Centre is the first support I've seen in a while for my theory that Type 1 diabetics have recoverable insulin producing capacity. Per the article on the Radio Netherlands Worldwide site,

11

Professor Roep discovered that people suffering from type 1 diabetes still have insulin-producing cells, albeit dormant. His discovery negates earlier research which concluded that these cells are completely absent in type 1 diabetes patients. If these cells can be reactivated the patient could be cured, even as long as 10 years after the original diagnosis was made.

Hot on the heels of the study by Professor Roep is another press release spotted in EurekaAlert! titled "Study finds some insulin production in long-term Type 1 diabetes". This is the second study in a week refuting the idea that a Type 1's beta cells are doomed as soon as the autoimmune attack begins.

Massachusetts General Hospital (MGH) research has found that insulin production may persist for decades after the onset of type 1 diabetes. Beta cell functioning also appears to be preserved in some patients years after apparent loss of pancreatic function.

My claims certainly sound more plausible with this kind of evidence. It's been a huge obstacle just to get people to believe that that a Type 1 pancreas is actually worth fighting for. Now maybe the argument can shift to HOW we can reactivate beta cells. Both the recent studies assume the need to develop a pharmacological agent of some sort. If you've read much of my story, you know that I defended and rebuilt my pancreas with diet, supplements, and a huge focus on stress reduction including acupuncture, yoga, and meditation. That proposition will still be a hard sell for years to come. But it seems a much closer goal now.

~~~

Fish Food For Thought

So you have a sick fish in an aquarium. The tank is looking pretty gross, so it's pretty obvious the poor little guy has been eating, drinking, and breathing some nasty looking water for a while.

The fish doctor comes over and takes a look. He does a blood test and returns with a Fishician's Order. He says, "There's no way this fish is getting better. He will develop multiple complications and die a premature death. You have to immediately begin daily injections to simulate the fresh water environment he's missing." When you sheepishly suggest that cleaning the tank might help, he just snorts condescendingly and leaves you with several samples of the stuff he wants you to start injecting poor Dory with. You watch from the door as he gets back in his Audi Quattro and dons a baseball cap with the same logo as the samples before backing out of the driveway.

(Metaphor key: Dory = your pancreas; aquarium = your body; dirty water = toxins from your lifetime eating of processed food; fish doctor = endocrinologist; injections = insulin; commercial bias and conflict of interest = exactly what it looks like)

WHAT'S YOUR STORY

Every day, in doctor's offices all around the world, people are hearing for the first time that they have diabetes. What happens next seems to vary. Shockingly, some are simply given a prescription for Metformin (a common oral medication) or for insulin supplies and sent on their way. Some Type 2's receive scolding about their weight. Many LADA's are misdiagnosed as Type 2's. Very few, even if they ask, get enough information.

The information newly diagnosed diabetics need to get includes what tests confirmed the diagnosis and what were the values. Some things are open to interpretation and you can't get a 2nd opinion, or form your own, if you don't know what the blood tests show. The *A1c* test is the primary indicator of high blood sugar levels. It's sometimes described as a 90 day average of your morning fasting finger prick self-tested blood glucose levels. I was advised to pay very little attention to the finger stick tests because of their extreme variability. Readings can change 30, 40, 50 points in seconds. The A1c is the only measure that counts in terms of tracking long-term progress. Any reading over 7 is going to suggest to a doctor that you might have diabetes, although you could be at that level for years without any real harm. My A1c was 11.1 when I was diagnosed, definitely over the line.

If your A1c is high for 3 months, and you're overweight, your doctor might look no further, assuming Type 2, and prescribe one or more of the oral medications that help bring blood sugar levels down. For a majority of diabetics, metformin (effective, cheap, and common) along with diet and activity improvements are enough to get back to normal.

If you're under age 20 and your A1c is high, your physician will suspect Type 1 and run tests for the antibodies that show up when your immune system attacks beta cells in your pancreas. If those come back positive, your doctor, or the endocrinologist she sends you to will order insulin for you. There will not be the slightest doubt in their mind that insulin is your only option. And if your pancreas is producing little or no insulin, they're right. You can't survive without it.

It's this question of how much insulin your pancreas is still producing that I raise my hand to ask. It determines whether you have time to try something else. It's not exact, but the C-peptide test is the usual measure for insulin production. Anyone suspected of having an autoimmune variety of diabetes should have this test as well as the antibody tests like GAD and IA-2 that can confirm that your pancreas is under attack.

Late-onset (Latent) Autoimmune Diabetes in Adults (LADA) is often misdiagnosed as Type 2 because traditionally, if someone over age 35 had a high A1c, Type 2 was the only known cause. My doctor suspected LADA because I was slim, with a relatively active lifestyle and met several other criteria that led him to test my C-peptide level. The problem with misdiagnosing a LADA as Type 2 is that if all they do is take the pills and clean up their diet, it'll work for a while but their pancreas will still be deteriorating until its function is so low it overcomes the positive effects of the metformin and healthier diet. They eventually have to take insulin because they're no longer producing enough. Sometimes, because of the misdiagnosis, they wait too long, and sustain more damage and complications than necessary.

Unfortunately, while it's good that awareness has made proper initial LADA diagnosis more likely, the result is that most LADA's are put on insulin immediately, just like traditional Type 1's. This is unfortunate because a LADA definitely has time before there's any risk of complications from his/her high blood sugar levels. A LADA's pancreas function decreases slowly over 2-12 years. For the first year at least, the oral medications will bring the A1c down. That *honeymoon*, through the time pills stop working and the A1c rises slowly to dangerous levels, is the time I used to try a natural or holistic approach.

WHY NOT JOIN THE CULT OF INSULIN

The knee-jerk prescription of insulin, which is now expanding even among pure Type 2's, is both maddening and discouraging.

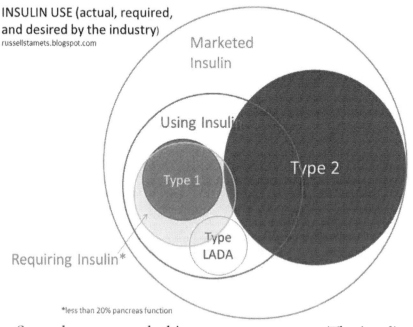

INSULIN USE (actual, required, and desired by the industry)
russellstamets.blogspot.com

Marketed Insulin

Using Insulin

Type 1

Type 2

Type LADA

Requiring Insulin*

*less than 20% pancreas function

Several groups push this extreme treatment. The insulin and insulin device industry are positively gleeful at the thought of hundreds of millions of diabetics world-wide dependent on their vials, syringes, pumps, and monitors. Healthcare professionals push it because anything holistic still sounds like *voodoo*, and in any case, it's easier to prescribe insulin and gain compliance than getting people to quit beer and doughnuts. And besides, the pharmaceutical reps seem pretty sincere and have good looking data. The other group that pushes insulin is the current users, including those that really require it, those who didn't question when they were ordered to, and those that chose it, preferring a daily shot in the stomach to giving up french fries.

~~~

the cult of insulin calls, seeks diabetics
straying into the valley of high A1c
they come, syringe in hand, acolytes of the easy way out
preaching "have your cake and eat it too"
teaching that "the bolus will balance your ongoing sin"
screeching, crow-like, at the heretic who chooses, instead
the hard climb out, scrabbling the canyon walls
reaching for a new life, independent, accountable
untethered to CGM, pump probe, or required refrigerator space

the heretic is no idiot!
he values his limbs, eyesight, and length of life
he merely questions the early, elective amputation
of a still functioning pancreas
the cult protests, "you whining needle-phobe, why limp?
That thing probably won't heal. Give it up.
Join our 24/7 party. Free hypos and constant calculations,
never a dull moment!"

the heretic reaches instead for the next handhold
patiently, consistently, lowering his A1c
with things like almonds, no batteries required
how boring! Using only force of will to cut the alcohol
and all the crap he so-long rained upon his body temple
and by degrees, to invite his detoxified vessel to trust him again,
and know that the decades long shock and awe campaign is over

the heretic will not pound his fist and demand, entitled
that his body resume the duties he once forfeited
the hysterical autoimmune attack, he knows
may only be called off in response to earnest non-violence,
a calm, sustained campaign of body-kindness, to which
the needle-jab and flow of foreign insulin is anathema.

WILL YOUR BODY EVER TRUST YOU AGAIN

This works both ways. You have to trust that your body is capable of healing itself and operating normally without foreign intervention. And your body has to trust you to not pour toxins into it or force it to function under the pressure of your stress.

It's funny how some of the most complex and difficult things can be said in few words.

This 2-way trust rebuilding is at the core of my approach. For us westerners, in particular, it's really hard to sit back in the buggy and choose an invisible, not-immediate, set of tools to accomplish something. Our whole psyche is in tune with doing something actively for a result right now. A pill, a shot, and instant results-- that's more like it! We don't have the patience, understanding, or faith that subtle, long-term, consistent actions can measurably affect our body. Simply choosing to not eat certain things over long periods of months, getting weekly acupuncture, and 15 minutes of meditation a day can't really cure a real, chronic disease, right? I wasn't sure when I started. But western medicine had only one, unacceptable road for me. Looking outside of that box was my only choice. I didn't abandon science. I was able to find studies supporting each component of my regimen, including acupuncture and meditation. The point here is that each of these things requires a commitment of time and trust if you're going to give it an honest try. It's a bet you have to go all-in for, unilaterally. You have to trust your body will respond to all this TLC long before it will calm down and trust that you've really changed your toxic ways.

I guess any real trust decision involves a gamble. Trusting enough to give this effort 100% risks what appears to be plenty. The rewards should be obvious, but what are the odds? Giving up alcohol and cherished foods. Doing *foo*

foo stuff like yoga and meditation? Working to change instincts and become a kinder person. All this means changing who you are. What if you like who you are now? If it doesn't work, what are you left with? Still sick and looking like the village idiot? These are all questions your *inner victim* will ask, cautioning, urging compromise, arguing against change.

Tell your victim to sit down and shut up.

WHAT ARE YOUR ISSUES

Zoomed out, you can look at anyone from a natural healing perspective and say they have two issues to deal with—diet and stress. The main goals of better glycemic control, consistent activity, and lower sustained stress are universal. Looking closer, everyone's solution will be some variation of a general recipe. One of your first tasks is to figure out where to focus. It'll seem less overwhelming when you realize that, of the whole list of factors to deal with, some are more of a problem than others. You don't have to expend as much energy on things that are already under control or that weren't a problem in the first place. If, for example, you don't drink, or drink very little, giving up alcohol won't be the big deal it is for someone like me. I drank an average of 2-3 beers 7 days a week for 25 years. All kinds of things become embedded in your lifestyle and persona with that kind of habit. The word habit is handy here. It makes you think of addiction. And addiction is what I realized most of us have to some things not usually classified that way. Studies are showing that fat and sugar stimulate the brain the same way that nicotine does. Even if you don't smoke, doesn't the craving for a doughnut seem a little too strong?

Before we even get to the specifics of a perfect diet and lifestyle, you should be able to highlight some things now that you know are going to be tough to quit or change. Just knowing the basic goals of a clean, lean and fresh diet, consistent activity, and minimal stress probably means putting a few things on the list right away. We'll talk more about which things should be quit cold turkey and which merely cut down. But you know nicotine, alcohol, and caffeine are on the list if you currently use them. No Starbucks? For some, like my wife, that would be a non-starter, no matter what the stakes. As for coffee, I'll preview now that it's one I've chosen to simply cut down drastically. Instead of all day long, I have a couple of cups of coffee in the morning, and then switch to de-caf (usually green tea) the rest of the day.

Besides those known addictive substances that might be on your list, you probably already know about the well-publicized enemies of diabetics—sugar and starch. We'll get to some fine points later, but added sugar (sucrose, the white stuff) is pretty much a poison just like a few people have been saying for some time now. If you're a sweet tea freak, or need it on cereal, or cook with it, this will be your issue. One quick note here: many processed foods you have to cut, like soda, are sweetened with *high fructose corn syrup,* a confusing name because it's just as bad as white sugar. Fructose, the stuff that's naturally in a piece of fruit, is OK. If your sweet tooth is big enough, it'll probably be your biggest issue. I can only tell you that the cravings will diminish. And for me fresh and dried fruit are as sweet as I'll ever desire.

When we talk about eliminating starches, it's the loss of the potato that makes me cry. I never met a potato I didn't like, especially with butter and cheese… and sour cream. At least the other starches, like white bread and white rice, have whole grain cousins that work great for me. And corn, chips or on the cob, doesn't seem to affect me. But the potato is huge. It and cheese vie for the top spot on my issues list.

Yup. I said cheese. We know we're going lean, so dairy has to go. Ouch! For me, cheese was a mainstay diet item like no other. I was a snob about only using or cooking with real butter, real sour cream, and full butter fat ice cream. Weight loss is not on my issue list, but in a cruel twist of fate, I've discovered that animal saturated fat has a huge effect on my blood sugar. At least I've always preferred my coffee black.

What other tough diet issues you can put on your specific list now? Do you hate to eat fresh green vegetables? That'll be tough. They are critical to the lean solution. One of the best ones for you, kale, tastes awful. But cooked, or dried, you don't taste it, and you'll still get the huge nutrient benefit. I've grown quite fond of some other greens. I cram all kinds of the cool lettuces we can get these days into my wraps and salads or piled on a sandwich.

How's your list so far? Cutting alcohol, caffeine, sugar, potatoes and eating green things would be a typical issue profile for the substance and diet areas. What about the *consistent activity* component? I think it's on nearly everybody's list. Who's got the time? Maybe nobody, but you'll have to make the time. It's as important as cutting the toxins out of your diet. More later, but the hint for now is that it doesn't have to be the full gym membership, massive sweat commitment thing. At least not for basic diabetes glycemic control. My minimum is 30 minutes of yoga/strength exercise in the morning, and at least 20 minutes of something in the afternoon. This might be a walk, mowing the lawn, chopping wood, whatever. I look for little opportunities all day long, like running up and down the stairs, or standing vs. sitting. You may have to double your activity time if weight loss is on your issue list. Remember, I'm one of the diabetics who are not trying to lose weight. For many of us, overcoming a lazy tendency, especially combined with other factors like living in a long-winter area, or being tied to a computer, is a top issue.

What about the stress side of the equation? And how the hell could you do anything about it anyway? Forget the second question for now. Break it up, see if there's any low hanging fruit. Family life, job, self-image, and personality type are all potential drivers for this critical factor. Is there an obvious standout contender here that you already know is killing you? For me, it was my job. I knew when I took my last one that the parts of management that have to do with messing with people's lives was against my nature. And boy was I right. The stress was exactly the dangerous kind my research has flagged. Long-term, persistent, stress triggered my LADA. Science's educated guess is that there's some kind of genetic predisposition that coupled with environmental factors like stress and bad diet gives the immune system the order to massacre the beta cells in the pancreas. I realized at the beginning that I had to attempt to fix the job situation… somehow. The other obvious factor for me was to learn to chill and cut down the number of things that piss me off. Every one of those *bang the steering wheel* road rage moments is food for the stress fiend. I wasn't a monster, but there was always a 50-50 chance if something went wrong, I'd have a little blow up. These were obvious targets for change. I've had some success changing my *fly off the handle* reactions. More detail later, but the acupuncture, meditation, yoga, and possibly certain supplements have modified me, surprisingly. If you'd asked me a year ago if I thought someone's basic instinct reaction could be changed, I'd have been positive the answer was no. But I had to try anyway. I should repeat a hundred times-- stress trumps all. You can change your diet and get active, but if you still have high, chronic stress levels, you won't succeed.

The good news is these stress areas overlap. You'll get synergistic bang for your buck. If you cut down the road rage moments, you'll cut down the snapping at your kids moments. If you're less of an asshole at home, family life improves.

Look honestly to find your stressor. Maybe you're the opposite of my arrogant, snappy tendency. Low self-image is just as stressful and defeating. This gets into the whole *can't be a victim* mantra I beat the drum about. Taking charge of yourself is just as important as not inappropriately taking charge of others. Every excuse crutch you use also feeds Stress, usually through the help of his good buddy Guilt.

Running out of space on your issues list? Don't get bummed. Go back and cross out all but the few biggest ones. Some are probably related and fixing the big one will cascade success into others. If you've ever done one of those personality surveys, the point here is similar—to cut the entire list of potential issues down to something manageable. You can't focus on everything at once. And you don't have to expend energy on things you already have under control.

Just thinking about modifying a horrible job or a bad marriage will probably cause stress in itself. There's no other way but to sound dramatic. The stress is killing you. If you don't do whatever it takes to fix or change it, you're proving you don't value your life.

HOW TO TRACK WITHOUT OBSESSION

Now that you've got a list of suspected, big picture issues, you need to start tracking. It's a crazy game that can cause stress in itself, but it's necessary. Keeping a record will confirm your suspicions, uncover unsuspected issues, and help you focus. It' will also confirm your success during the long 3 month periods between your A1c lab tests.

Blood sugar, or blood glucose, whatever you want to call it, is the all-consuming focus for all diabetics. How often to measure, when, and exactly what any particular number means, are not standardized answers even within the Diabetes Establishment. The answers are definitely different depending on whether you are using insulin or not.

No matter what the arguments are for the efficacy of the finger stick blood glucose test, you have to use it and test constantly if you're injecting insulin or using a pump. Insulin acts like gasoline on hot coals. You never know exactly how high the flare will be or how long. Read the diabetes blogs and community sites and you'll see the roller coaster ride described over and over again by Type 1's who inject, then their number goes too low, then they eat to bring it up, then they test and test and test and the cycle goes on. Insulin users who don't mind the cyborg life have some interesting alternatives to the syringe and the finger stick these days. The two tools that have people most excited are the insulin pump and the continuous glucose monitor (CGM). The pump has been around a while. It's true I don't like needles, but this thing makes me cringe too. You strap a cell phone sized box somewhere that hopefully won't show under your clothes (like in the small of your back) and stick the tube from it into somewhere like your stomach. You fill it's hopper up with insulin, dial in an amount for it to deliver, and then instead of injecting so often with a syringe, you dial it up or down based on meals or when you feel dizzy from a low. The *site* or place you stick the tube has to be changed periodically. Apparently there are various irritations and other complications to keep you busy with these things. Insulin users swear by them though, citing major quality of life improvements.

The CGM is relatively new development that many insulin users are scrambling to get. It's another battery powered device you wear around all the time with another probe you stick into yourself. It's basically a 24/7 finger stick test. You can glance at the sunglasses case-sized device clipped to your belt anytime you want and see your current blood sugar level as it perpetually races up and down the scale from meal to meal. Now, in a movie or a business meeting, in addition to forgetting to turn off a pager or a cell phone, the forgetful cyborg diabetic can announce, via an exciting series of beeps, that he or she has a blood sugar level that is too high or too low. The most advanced of these battery encrusted airport security nightmares will have the pump and the CGM working together, with the pump responding to the meter to automatically control the flow of insulin. All that's needed now for the ultimate diabetic nerd nirvana is a wrist mounted vending machine that could drop a piece of fudge in your hand whenever your blood sugar is too low.

All joking aside, the fact is that the insulin user must test, before and after meals, and whenever else his/her wackily adjusted system dictates. That's another world, one I hope to never have great familiarity with. Because if you're like me, and don't' take insulin, testing has an entirely different goal and timeframe. One possibility is that you *never* use the finger stick test and focus solely on the every 3 month (or every six months if you're under control)

A1c test. The strict evidence-based medicine guys say it's the only proven measure of blood glucose levels. This could be the least stressful strategy, but it requires a hefty measure of drive and consistency and faith. That's a lot to ask, especially in the early days after diagnosis when fear, guilt, and a cloud of unknowns hang over you.

I decided to use a daily, single, morning fasting finger stick blood glucose test as part of my tracking process in spite of the reliability questions. I'm kind of a numbers guy by nature and wanted immediate feedback. As it turns out, the 90 day average of my morning fasting numbers matches my A1c pretty closely which makes it a meaningful measure. In a new development, there are finger stick A1c tests hitting the market now. These might make sense for those that want to make daily testing part of their tracking.

Along with the graph of my blood sugar levels each day, I note everything I eat, what exercise or activity I have for the day, what stress incidents (good or bad) happen, my weight, and anything relevant like starting or stopping a supplement, or an acupuncture appointment. I keep just enough detail to be useful, but not so much that I can't keep up with it each day. In the early days, when my blood sugar was swinging between 150 and 250 or more, it sometimes seemed impossible that anything useful could ever be deciphered from the information I recorded.

But I did learn from it. In early Spring of 2011, I had stabilized a little, but I would still have some kind of a spike over 190 at least every 10 days. I would always look at what I'd eaten or done, or gotten stressed about the day before. Sometimes it was obvious. One of the biggest clues came on May 1 when my morning reading was 213, not great. Nothing stood out in the log of diet and activity from the day before. Dinner had been a Cuban pulled pork sandwich at a favorite pub in Loveland. It had seemed a reasonable choice-- protein, not a huge portion. But this time it caught my eye. I'd had the identical meal about 12 days before, the night before a spike of 196. I was sure there was a connection, but it eluded me until May 15 with my next spike of 215. Dinner before that was pot roast. How could that be bad, great protein with vegetables? I googled and finally found a likely culprit. I found a study showing that animal saturated fat caused blood sugar levels to rise. The usual diabetes diet warnings only mention this kind of fat in the context of weight loss. This is one of the only pieces of evidence I've seen connecting it with blood sugar directly. Since keeping weight *on* has been my issue through all this, I thought dairy, pot roast, and pulled pork were a great combination of protein and some fat to keep my weight up.

When I checked back in my tracking log, I found other spikes where animal saturated fat was a suspect. Cheesy nachos, whole milk in a latte, bacon, all looked like problems. Strangely enough, a grilled steak is fine. Plant fats, like olive oil have no effect. As soon as I cut out all dairy, and all beef or pork that was cooked in its own juices (not grilled), I saw significant improvement in my numbers.

Another clue proven by my tracking to be correct was eating dinner early. I'd seen a study, also confirmed by my nutritionist, suggesting I shouldn't eat anything after 8. My log showed a correlation with late dinners or snacks and a higher number the next day. I always have dinner finished before 8 now and I'm sure it's one ingredient in my success.

Tracking doesn't have to be a chore. Keep it simple or you won't stick with it. Keep the minimum of information that you think you can use. I don't track quantities of food, for example. For a while I took a snapshot of my plates with my smart phone to show my nutritionist what I was eating. She was impressed!

The Excel sheet I use has a row for each day. My columns include: date, meter reading, eats, exercise, stress, other, and weight. My "eats" entries are a shorthand.

Yesterday for example it reads "rye/pb/oatm/cinn/wlnt/cinn/blu/rasbry, salmon/bellpeppr/green onion wrap, salsa/chips/beef jerky/apple" The commas separate breakfast, lunch, and dinner. I don't note all the almonds, sunflower seeds, or other between meal snacks. The stress column notes good and bad effects. For me, it usually includes meditation. If something lousy happened, I note it here too.

Tracking is a fine balance. One of the main benefits of my approach is to reach a point where diabetes has minimal impact on the way you live and enjoy each day. That means not spending much time with things like tracking. But it's hard, especially in the scary early days, not to obsess over it. All I can say is that beyond the minimal logging I've described, any additional time is better spent taking a walk, doing yoga or meditating for 15 minutes.

I do spend too much time staring at the graph of my morning fasting Blood Sugar measurements. The trend line is my crystal ball to the past, present, and future of how I fare in my battle with diabetes. I can draw that trend line in drastically different ways. Which way do I choose at any given time? To appear positive, of course! This day last October is a good example. By changing the polynomial order of the Excel trend line tool, I can tell different stories, although only for recent times. Long term, it's less flexible.

Trend Scenario for 10/16/2011 using polynomial order "3" This would be the pessimistic view that after the drastic drops in July/August, I'm trending back up to soon be above the *diabetic* line again and toward required insulin use:

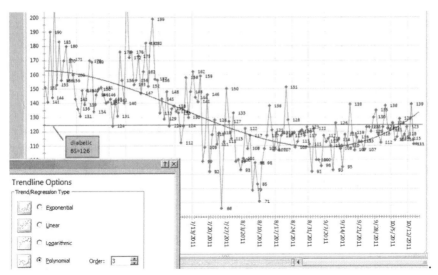

Trend Scenario for 10/16/2011 using polynomial order "5". This would be the probably overly optimistic tea leaf reading. The spin for this view would be that after a little bump from the stress of the initial going public online with my story, the last couple of days show me trending back down:

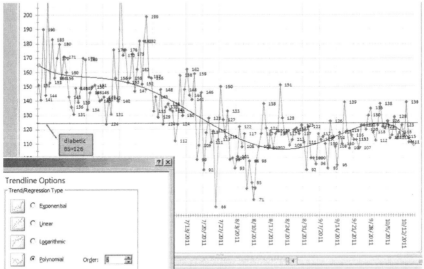

Trend Scenario for 10/16/2011 using polynomial order "2". In true Goldilocks fashion, the middle of the road interpretation is my choice today. Little uptrend yes, but explainable, and sweetened with the observation that

daily swings are drastically dampened and stabilized. Yes!
This is the view that the *Russell News Channel* will go with
today:

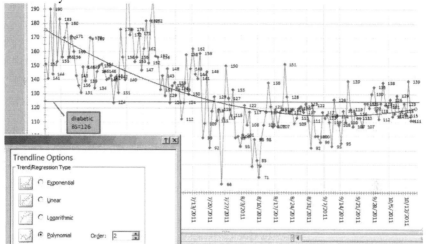

WHO ELSE IS ALONG FOR THE RIDE

I hope you're not alone. Even the strongest among us couldn't manage this without help. There are three categories of people most diabetics will have around them during this incredible journey. There's the paid group of healthcare professionals, including your physician and maybe an endocrinologist. My acupuncturist/nutritionist has become such a close friend; she's also part of the second group of those that choose to help me. This group includes friends who could keep distance from the *diabetes thing*, but are interested. It also includes the active Diabetes Online Community (DOC) and *live* groups that exist to support diabetics throughout the country. The third group includes your husband, wife, kids, parents, partner, roommate, and anyone else who has no choice but to ride with you. They didn't ask for this and, although it's a challenge to look up and around often enough, you better figure it out. This group is your biggest asset— or the cause of your defeat if you neglect them.

It's quite a mindset change for many of us to think of our doctor as our hired hand, paid to serve us, and accountable. The culture has been to treat them unquestioningly, like a priest. Would I have questioned my physician when I was diagnosed if he'd insisted that I begin insulin immediately? That would have changed everything. Fortunately, his interpretation of facts and individual reading of me, allowed my questions. The answers to those questions prompted me to look east. The western side of medicine is absolutely uniform in its belief that *autoimmune=irreversible*. Simple as that.

No smart eastern practitioner will irresponsibly guarantee a specific result, but every one of them believes that every body process can at least be acted upon with... let's say *statistically* time proven techniques. It's a fascinating mix of precise and vague. Precise, perhaps, in terms of intricate body energy point maps (i.e. for acupuncture), and yet vague in our reckoning when noting a fact like the pancreas may not be identified specifically, but it's part of a system with liver and spleen. Much about this way of thinking appeals to me. Kind of like the mix between astrophysics and creative writing that were my majors in college. I like eastern trained practitioners because the connections they make, especially in terms of problem solving, are intuitive, broad, and interdisciplinary.

The first conversation I had with Jane, my acupuncturist, was eye-opening. I hadn't read much at that point about acupuncture or any of the underlying theory, but what she said made so much sense. A huge result of that first discussion was to quit alcohol. As I provided a volume of diet, activity and stress detail, I told her about the changes I'd made already since diagnosis, including cutting out the rum and most of the beer and switching to a couple of glasses of wine. She said, "the liver and the pancreas are a system. Any stress on the liver is stress on the pancreas. Even though your liver is fine, you should quit alcohol to give your pancreas the best chance to heal." "Oh great", I thought. I really could've used that particular vice to help get through this thing. But I knew she was right. It made too much sense. Even though it was Friday, with cocktail hour anticipated, I went home and had tea. It made so much sense I didn't even try to hold it at bay with any argument like the fact that my physician Fabio thought the cut back to wine was a reasonable strategy. Of course, I'd have been a hypocrite if I hadn't quit. I was scared enough to be really serious. I stuck by a vow to try ANYTHING that I thought was within reason. Jane's simple logic on this question far more than passed the bar of *within reason*. That's one of many decision points sparked by Jane's interest and expertise. The acupuncture, supplement research, and nutrition counseling are critical. We've really had collaboration over the last year that has shaped this regimen. I don't think there's any question that you want some authentic eastern-mindedness on your bus.

I asked Jane how she thought my story applied to everyone else:

Russell's medical situation, an interesting iteration of adult onset latent autoimmune diabetes, seems fairly unique. Even more rare, and against most medical advice, Russell chose a grassy, untrammeled path in lieu of the insulin superhighway. Not accepting insulin as his first line of treatment thankfully thrust Russell back on himself as his main healer. I'm sure this process has been somewhat lonely for him. There is no defined, discrete roadmap, no sure prognosis, and few sympathetic doctors (though he did find one). This "thanks, but no" required a very thorough investigation of the path that led him to this troubling diagnosis and a full accounting of some possible lifestyle transgressions. Though Russell has chosen the more challenging approach, I am hoping he is not unique in the way he has taken full responsibility for his present and past life choices. The changes he has made are at present a winning combination that have stabilized his blood sugars, and lowered his A1c, positive movement toward decelerating or stopping the progression of LADA. The power of these changes cannot be underestimated and our message is that they are all within our grasp. And the more you do, the better you do.

Chinese medicine, which I practice, is heavily weighted toward having people recognize basic universal, natural laws regarding living and health consequences - laws that if disregarded short term can lead to minor health problems: If you're not getting enough good quality sleep you may be more susceptible to an "evil pathogen" entering the exterior of your body such as "wind cold or wind heat". That "evil" looks a lot like our cold or flu. The evil remains on the surface of the body and does not become entrenched at deeper levels. We quickly recover. However, ignoring natural laws over a longer time can result in more egregious consequences - much harder to rectify. For instance, if we are overtaxing ourselves at work (or play) over years, and eating poorly (you know who you are), our basic life energy reserves become depleted, our life force or "qi" is deficient and possibly stagnant like a stream in late fall or even a swamp. Disease can develop at much deeper levels and become lodged.

Clearly Russell had gone beyond a simple flu. Unbeknownst to himself he had been shirking his responsibilities to his body for years. He had been eating far from the "whole" side of foods, working very hard, perhaps drinking too much, not moving his body like it wanted to. And for a long time he got away with it. He felt healthy actually. (Ringing any bells?) But damage was done and his particular make up decided his pancreas might be sacrificed. Still, Russell is on a continuum of disease, for neither has his pancreas failed him, nor has his insulin sensitivity run aground. His body is still fertile ground for change and hope. Many of us are somewhere on this continuum, maybe with a diagnosis or still in the developing stages of disease. In Chinese medicine we say that "all disease starts at the qi level". We might have strange, intermittent symptoms that doctors are mystified by, where no lab test can detect any known disease. We look good on paper but feel "off", not ourselves. That's qi level stuff. That would be the perfect time to start changing lifestyle, but we and our health system have not been trained to intervene in our own lives until something is really wrong. So we go beyond qi level. Now we're in trouble. Now we have a diagnosis and probably interventions, i.e., medications. Russell got into this level of trouble, and maybe you're reading this book because you are too.

But since Russell made the changes you will read about he feels the healthiest he has felt in years, which leads me to believe he wasn't actually feeling that great after all. I'll pause here so you can ask yourself how you're feeling these past months or years....Point made.

The message Russell wants to convey is that he doesn't want you to be alone in your quest for improved health no matter your situation. And he doesn't want to be alone either.
In my experience Russell has delved more deeply into his mind, body and spirit than any health practitioner can ever even dream of; he has been more compliant and vigilant than I could even hope for myself and his rewards have been obvious, inspiring and downright astounding. It's certainly a daily challenge for him, but one that addresses the root cause of his dis-ease and is thereby ultimately satisfying.

I'm pretty lucky that Jane chose this puzzle to work on. Her skilled acupuncture alone is a major component of my success, but having someone with a professional eye to scrutinize supplement choices and dosages with an eye to my overall balance is priceless.

The group of those along for your diabetes ride that do it voluntarily are another indispensable source of information and support. Friends you had from before diagnosis and patient advocates you discover online have free advice and perspectives not available from your paid professionals. Of course you have to take it with a grain of salt. You're in charge, as always. Nobody can make a decision that's right for you, except you. But these guys could save your life. No matter how self-sufficient you are, hearing stories from other diabetics makes it impossible to claim you're alone.

I have to admit I avoided the Type 1 diabetic discussion forums for a long time. It made me sick to my stomach. So much of the discussion is centered on the 24 hour ordeal of messing around with insulin. Especially when I still thought that was my fate. Most of the Type 1 diabetic community is consumed with the taking and management of this crazy drug. They swing in frustration from high to low, wagging the dog. I just couldn't look at it at first. Now that it appears I'm not on that road, I read some of it, trying to engage with these folks, trying to learn. Some people I've talked to that were already insulin users have been able to safely cut it back after trying the kind of diet, supplement, and stress changes that I'm detailing in this book. That was surprising. I initially thought only the newly diagnosed would be able to leverage their remaining pancreas function to reverse the disease.

So use the diabetes community for the wealth of information, and the shoulders to cry on, that it contains. As always, filter information, and don't get sucked in to the depressing, victimized place that many diabetics live in.

Last, and most importantly, I'll remind you to keep a constant watch on how your closest traveling companions are faring. Husband, wife, partner, son, daughter, or whoever's in the house with you, day to day. These guys are unpaid, involuntary partners in this thing that's happened to you. Diabetes has happened to them too. They're sometimes referred to as Type 3. Parents of diabetic kids, in particular, have an intense experience of handling every day to day detail without actually feeling a high or low or needle stick.

You may come out of all of this better, with stronger relationships, but not before some serious testing. Your situation won't be the same as mine in this respect either, so my challenges, setbacks, and victories are only examples of infinite possibilities. One thing probably true for all is that whatever weak spots you have in your psyche and in your relationship with your family will be exaggerated, at least at first. When people are scared, they become hyper-reactive. After diagnosis, everybody in your immediate vicinity is scared, same as you. "How will this affect our plan to retire to a sailboat in a couple of years? Will the kids develop this too? How are we all going to change our diet? Will we ever get insurance again?" In my case, my wife also had to wonder, "if he was so self-centered before, how bad is it going to get now that so much of the day to day revolves around his diabetes?" And, "if he has to quit his job because of the stress, how will we survive?"

If you and your spouse/partner do nothing but loop these questions non-stop, you're screwed. The stress from it will pour gas on either your autoimmune pancreas attack (Type 1) or the inflammation of your insulin resistance (Type 2). And your loved one will likely get sick from the stress as well. So don't go there. This is where you need to have already jettisoned your victim. Your victim will invite you to wallow in fear and indecision if he's still with you. You won't be able to take the positive lead that you MUST. Your complete control of your recovery means that no other cheery individual can lead you moping (or kicking and screaming) down the right path. You have to sincerely exude hope and positive energy and inspire your family. You have to lead them out of the waiting room and into the fresh air and the excitement of an "I wonder what's down that path?" kind of adventure. You owe it to them. Your goal is to say "Diabetes is the best thing that ever happened to me" *and mean it.*

That's the tricky part. It's not a matter of a stiff upper lip. You have to actually get there, believing your Mary Poppins preaching. How? I'm still working on it. One answer is that there are so many benefits from the changes I've made, beyond just the curing of the diabetes. Having a body this healthy and a mind that's calmer, kinder, more balanced is an incredible payoff for all the work that went into this. When I realized it wasn't about trying to get back to the state I was in before diabetes, my cheerleading made the leap to heartfelt and gained conviction. When my A1c started dropping due to my efforts, I saw this whole thing wasn't about trying to catch up to my prior path and just accept some lost time and lifelong quality of life compromise like taking insulin. This was about leapfrogging to a better life. I have understood this to be true before my family could see it. But they trust my optimism enough to put most of the fear aside and move forward with me. Managing my stress is connected with every single aspect of this story. If I can't do it, I can't be the sincerely optimistic leader and I can't maintain healthy, sustainable relationships with my family or my body.

"Judge Not" is the title of an early Bob Marley tune. This simple two-word rule might be all you need in your battle with stress. Stress kills. If not directly, it's indicted for multiple chronic inflammatory diseases. Stress is trickier than any other component of healing. You can't eliminate it by conscious choice. Understanding it intellectually doesn't really help. You can't will yourself to chill. And the real kicker is that even if you don't feel stressed, your body can still be suffering damage from it.

Libraries full of books, medical professional buildings full of psychologists, ashrams full of gurus, and a multi-billion dollar pharmaceutical industry all provide answers to the stress problem. I would charitably assume that every one of these must've actually provided a solution for somebody at some time. But I know for a fact that any sustainable solution involves some proactive work by the stressee. And among all the exercises, meditation practices, and the rest, the most powerful tip is probably the simple mandate to quit being judgmental.

I was sorry, in a way, when it became apparent how critical this is. I've always been quite good at judging others. It was a skill to be proud of, maybe even one of those self-defining pillars. But no more— at least not the proud or defining part. It'll probably take years, if ever, before I can say I never slip. Still, 90% less judgmental has huge payoffs. It's cut the angry, sad, pained, vindictive, and all such ugly moments that arise from it. Those moments are prime stress drivers. I'm saying you can't directly will a reduction in stress; but, you can consciously begin to limit your judgmental tendencies. A little less fist pounding when cut off in traffic will, in itself, be well received by your head and gut. If, simultaneously, you begin treating your body with some respect in terms of what you put in it, you can spark a beneficial feedback loop. Because a less stressed body is calmer at a cellular or gut level and less likely to suggest fist pounding.

My wife and daughters were already eating pretty well before my diabetes. Chalk part of this up to their perpetual dieting, but they ate reasonable amounts of fruits and vegetables and much less processed food than most, including me. It drove them crazy that I could eat so badly and stay skinny. And then, of course, we found out I had a different price than weight to pay for eating the great American diet. The moderate changes I made for the first year and a half brought me more in line with how Kathy and the girls were eating. So I'd actually eat the fish dish Kathy made instead of turning up my nose and making a burrito swimming in a couple of pounds of cheese to eat instead. But at the beginning of 2011 the tables turned completely. Along with cold turkey on alcohol, my all-out effort to beat LADA meant keeping a pretty extreme eye on everything, with drastic cuts to starches, non-whole grain carbs, and eventually animal saturated fats. The restrictions on how late I could eat dinner and keeping pounds of snackable almonds around at all times also created stress for Kathy. How was she supposed to prepare two different meals? Where were all these crazy ideas coming from? Was Russell really obsessing out of control over this stuff? Why can't he just sit down and have a glass of wine with me? All of these questions have reasonable answers. But taken altogether, they're overwhelming. That usual, unsatisfying answer, *time*, is the one here as well.

The one thing you absolutely can't do to your family is ask them to do it too. Sure, it'd be easier for you if all the cookies and chips were just gone from the house. But it's not fair. There's enough danger of resentment without forcing them to change their lifestyles. You need to just worry about yourself. It's probably good for you to live within reach of fresh baked brownies anyway. They eventually become more of a regular, visible affirmation of your positively changed self than the destructive siren call they might be at first. Just keep the almonds and fruit handy.

It's worth noting that at this point, Kathy and the girls are healthier than they were previously too. I'm sure it's partly from seeing the results on me and partly from less processed food being in the house, but they've voluntarily changed their habits over this last year. There's that *change* word again. Everybody's changed. Yikes! We were OK before. How different a person have I become? In frustrated moments, Kathy has says she wishes she had the old me back. I try not to be hurt. I wondered from the beginning what kind of difference cutting something as core as drinking out of my life would make. It's interwoven at every social level, from Kathy and my Sunday morning mimosas to every single small or large social gathering in our typical American life. I've always thought teetotalers were *off* just a bit. Nice enough, but missing a vital connecting tie with the rest of us regular Joe's.

Kathy's wishing for the *old me* comment though is usually referring to another perception of change in me. At times during this, she has seen me as starting from an already pretty self-centered place and moving much further into a zone of self-absorption. Asked if she thinks it's *all about me* at these times, she'd swear "Hell yes!" It's true you have to look inside pretty intently as you disassemble yourself looking for the places where things like alcohol and anger are connected. Then you have to rebuild with the parts that are left and see how you run. I have to trust Kathy when she says I got worse during that process about not looking beyond myself. My own perceptions are that I made significant improvement. Go figure! One reason for the discrepancy might be a form of inertia. During a short period of time I altered my anger reflex. It was one of the most obvious stress reducing targets I could see. The acupuncture and meditation, and possibly even my less-inflamed cells were quickly making me less inflamed and likely to fly off the handle. From Kathy's perspective, decades old patterns of conversation and emotion between us were suddenly altered. My failure to rise to anger at a moment that all history says I would was a significant change. My attempt at measured, calmer responses must've seemed disengaged? Or condescending? Who knows? It doesn't really matter. All that matters is that even with your hands full of yourself, you need to look up. And remember that perception is all there is. Your loved ones' perceptions, that is. Your intent doesn't count. I hate that fact. But it's the most proven pearl of wisdom I can offer.

HOW MANY TIMES IS "JUST THIS ONCE"

Where exactly are the hard lines drawn in the sand? When is compromise not equal to defeat? Which rules have any flexibility? The unhelpful answer would be a simple "it depends." Figuring out which rules you can bend depends on several factors: your trickiest addictions; your goals; your personality; and your attitude to name a few. Some of the less individual considerations include whether some food or activity has an immediate effect on blood sugar, or is more of a long term goal. And you may tweak and adjust over time. I was very strict with my *rules* for the first six months. Since then I have experimented with a few compromises.

Alcohol is a good example of a tweak. It's a big deal. There are mental and social issues in addition to the physical concerns. It has no immediate effect on BS, at least not on the next-morning fasting test that I use. But it's definitely one of those slippery slope possibilities for me. I definitely needed the 6 month cold turkey to break the mental addiction as well as give the liver/pancreas team as low stress a sabbatical as possible. But even with the physical and mental desire pretty much gone, the social pressure makes it constantly a contender for experimenting with exceptions. What I decided to a few months ago was to allow myself to share a bottle of champagne with my wife (or whoever). Champagne occasions don't usually occur more than once a month. And they are usually psychologically potent occasions. Not participating in that ritual for celebrations is a very visible reminder of the *diabetes beast* and the changes it represents. My goal to minimize its impact and visibility elevated this to a level making alcohol worth a modest experiment.

Examples of no compromise foods include potatoes, cheese, and any kind of pastry or cake. With exceptions like trying one (and only one) of Kathy's French fries when we're out to eat, or one bite of key lime pie, or a miniscule amount of lean cheese grated on a salad, I'll remain strict with these things indefinitely. Not a single soda this past year, or a baked potato has past my lips. I actually dreamed about a baked potato a few nights ago. It had sour cream and butter on it, neither of which have I had any quantity of on this diet. I'm sure there's been butter or cream cooked into something I've eaten in a restaurant. I don't grill our servers on the ingredients of every dish. That's one of those distasteful, visibly diabetic things I decline to do. I make my best guesses in restaurants and haven't had a serious spike from a mystery ingredient yet.

My next chapters will finally detail food, supplements, and rules. My goal is to set the stage and answer a few questions before you start to sweat the menu plans. Did I say menu plans? No. Even as a list-making, detail kind of guy I could never do the whole carb-counting, serving-weighing thing that seems to be the core of most diets. I want simple, clear-cut choices. I want to know generally what I can eat, when I need to eat it, and what very few things might be negotiable. I want to be able to go out to eat wherever the group is going and know I can find something on the menu I can eat. If I have any doubt, I'll snack on my beef jerky and dried mango before we go. But the fact is, there's some kind of grilled chicken or salmon salad I can eat almost anywhere these days. Not that extremely challenging occasions don't arise. I was in New Bern, NC this summer and went with relatives to a place where the pre-dinner bread/rolls they brought out were croissants drizzled in honey. As usual for North Carolina, there is no iced tea that's not sweet tea. And, unfortunately, every single one the beautiful cuts of grilled meat this place had that I otherwise could've eaten were prepared with their signature butter infused and basted sauce. As long as your victim is long gone, these occasions are more humorous anecdote than pain. I do find it really interesting these days to watch other people drink a lot.

Rules I attempt to never break, not even once, include not eating after 8pm. This has made a huge difference in my numbers, especially as part of the changes I made to eat regularly throughout the day. Never skip breakfast. If you're travelling, this is another place a backpack full of almonds, beef jerky, dried fruit, and maybe some low-sugar granola bars can keep you compliant.

I'm also strict about my supplements. I still don't know exactly which ones are making the biggest difference, but Jane and I made our best guess, good results have happened, and I'm loathe to change the routine without good reason.

Regular activity is also non-negotiable. This is where the fact that my definition of activity doesn't have to include sweat or a gym makes this rule maintainable even while traveling or even when you have a cold. The more the better, but I have an absolute minimum of 30 minutes of yoga/strength exercises with the Wii fit, or a walk, or mowing the lawn (walk-behind mower, not riding). Generally I want at least 20 minutes of something active in addition to the yoga.

I can say that the stress control rules are strictly inflexible, but there is the question of how much is within your control. You can make the time to meditate for 15 minutes every day. It's hard, seems like such a waste of time on busy days. But who knows, it may be the most effective tool in this plan to reverse the autoimmune attack. Others have tried even stricter diet and exercise routines than I advocate and still had their pancreas function decline steadily. Something I'm doing in addition to the diet and activity is reviving my pancreas. It has to be either the supplements or the yoga and meditation or the combination. Since the autoimmune attack is by far the most important goal for anyone on the Type 1 half of the spectrum, it seems foolhardy to compromise any of these few ingredients that might be achieving it. Those on the Type 2 side of things may have to substitute getting the weight off for the most critical goal. That'll mean even lower carb intake and probably more of a fight to stay uncompromised on diet.

WHAT TO EAT

So why in the world is the most important thing, THE ACTUAL DIET, placed this far into the book? Because it's not the most important piece of my plan. Should I put that in CAPS too? The diet is critical, but it's no more important than the head game. The diet alone won't work if your stress levels cancel out its benefit. Even this diet is as much about attitude as the details. I'm finally going to list the rules, but it's not about memorizing and blindly following rules. It's about understanding the big picture and knowing the logic of the goals. This keeps it much simpler to figure out what to do, and much easier to hold steady as a rock when the cheesecake tray floats by. This diet philosophy can drastically improve your glycemic control and set the stage for the supplement, activity, and stress-reduction components to perform the other miracle of stopping the autoimmune attack.

I want you to know what classes of food you can eat and in what general proportions. After a few weeks of carbs and sugar trying to lure you back, your body will take care of most of the work. You won't have to count every morsel you eat. You're just going to eat good stuff, spread out throughout the day, with nothing after 8pm. Those of you that have weight loss as a goal will have a slightly lower proportion of whole grains and nuts than those of us that need more good fat and a few more carbs to keep weight on.

You can use tools like a Glycemic Index (GI) table to get started, but take it with a grain of salt. It's not an exact science because there are so many individual differences. It's important to track what you eat and look for foods that spike your blood sugar. Some of these may not rate badly on the GI table even though your body reacts adversely to them.

I don't use the tables. It's still too complicated for me. I want simple rules that make it easy when I'm looking at a menu or shopping in the grocery store. I don't rate potato dishes differently for example. The GI table rates a baked potato as worse than fries or sweet potato which are worse than potato chips. That's too tricky for a life-long potato lover like me. I have just cut them all out. Thank God corn chips don't raise my BS at all. Without chips and salsa, the world would be far less rosy.

My diet is lean, uses very little that's processed (comes in cans), has lots of fruit and vegetables and nuts. Lots o nuts!

~~~

How are your nuts?

wonderful walnuts in my oatmeal at 7
first fist-full of almonds with banana around 10
salty sunflower seeds suffuse lunch's wrap at 1
more almighty almonds with dried mango at 3
perhaps pistachios arriving home at 5
or curry cashews for cocktail hour
and walk the wild side with wasabi almonds in dinner's salad

I love my nuts!

~~~

Let's walk through a typical day of what I eat and drink to give you an idea of what this idea looks like:

Breakfast—just like they always said (and I used to ignore), it's the most important meal of the day. My only caffeine is my 1-2 cups of morning coffee. Two pieces of some very whole grainy bread, toasted with peanut butter. I like both the Sprouted Rye and Sprouted Barley I pick up at

Natural Grocer. Next I have a bowl of old-fashioned oatmeal, with a liberal amount of cinnamon and walnuts. The cinnamon has long been suggested to help blood sugar control. The walnuts are some extra good fat to keep meat on my skinny bones. You can forego them if you're trying to lose. I would've sworn I could never eat oatmeal without the brown sugar I always used to use, but I don't miss it. The cinnamon is awesome. I also get some sweetness along with the oatmeal in the form of blueberries, raspberries, blackberries, or strawberries. I almost always have at least a couple of varieties on hand and have at least a handful a day. These berries get a lot of press these days. They are flavonoids that are apparently beneficial in several ways. Eggs are great. I might have them instead of the oatmeal. Just cook the in olive oil or with a spray or anything that's not butter. If I have bacon, which I love, it's turkey bacon these days. I would have turned up my nose and scoffed at the thought before, but cooked crisp, it's perfectly satisfying to me with eggs, or in a wrap salad)

I was never a big milk drinker, but since that's part of many breakfasts, I might as well mention a huge cut from my old diet and the reason I mention turkey bacon. I cut animal saturated fat almost entirely from my diet which includes all dairy. This is one of those things that's not standard with other diets. What's interesting about it is that while I can't eat pot roast, I can eat a steak from the grill. For beef and pork, it's something about when they're cooked in their own juices, like many stews or chilies or the Cuban pulled pork sandwich that tipped me off. And the fat in butter, milk, and cheese, falls in the same category. It's too bad, not only because of how huge a part of my old diet cheese was, but because it would have been a great way to keep weight on. You'll have to see if this is true for you.

If I'm on the road and can't get my standard breakfast, I'll have fresh or dried fruit, a low carb/sugar granola bar, and maybe a fruit drink. Make sure you start looking at the nutrition labels to find the lower carb and sugar items. Granola bars, for instance, vary hugely.

Mid-morning Snack—many days, I'll have a banana and some almonds around 10:30. This was more critical when I was still taking oral diabetes medications that could lower blood sugar enough at times to make you lightheaded if it had been more than a few hours since a meal. Notice I don't mention much in the way of quantities. That's because if you're only eating good stuff, you can eat until you're full.

Lunch—a whole wheat tortilla wrap with whatever was the grilled lean meat from last night is common. Steak, chicken, salmon, pork roast and lettuce, onion, maybe a few kalamata olives and sunflower seeds are common wrap fillings for me. Occasionally topped with a low fat, low sugar dressing, but the flavors in most of my ingredients are usually plenty. If I'm still hungry I'll have an apple or a kiwi. If I'm out sailing I might eat just dried mango and almonds and one of those healthy granola bars. Eating out is easy. There's almost always a salad that's acceptable.

Afternoon Snack—more nuts and fruit

Dinner—all the things to avoid have been mentioned, like potatoes and white flour pasta and white rice and cheese, and non-grilled beef and pork. The *OK* list includes the wide world of fresh and cooked vegetables and BEANS, wonderful beans. Another thing I would have said "no way" to before diabetes would be the thought of using ground turkey for chili or tacos. Turns out it's great. As spicy as those dishes are it doesn't really make any difference.

It's worth mentioning here that Kathy and I have started getting as much organic as we can. There's now some evidence that the various hormones and other trace toxins contribute to diabetes and other inflammatory and autoimmune diseases. It's more expensive, but we spend some of the beer savings on organic vegetables and pasture fed ground beef. It might be all in our head, but the green chile cheeseburgers made from that stuff on the grill are fantastic. Yes, I said CHEESEburger. The only dairy I have these days is a little sharp cheddar on a green chile cheeseburger.

There are some great synergies for a better world with this diet. Reducing processed or packaged foods as much as possible is greener. Shopping more often for fresh meat and vegetables is different than the huge Cost Co stock up run. Everybody says it costs more to eat well. But, of course, that's not figuring in green or health savings.

Other *what to eat/what not to eat* notes include quitting alcohol. If you're a social drinker this one is tough mentally. It's getting more common, but people still tend to think non-drinkers are a little odd. I've found a couple of non-alcoholic beers that actually taste good. They are pricey, so I don't drink but a fraction of what I used to consume in regular beer. But with certain meals, or when around other people drinking, it's nice to have a cold one in your hand.

A note about fruit—other diets are all over the board on this one. What I've found is that any fruit, and as much of it as I want is good for me. I see no blood sugar effects from fructose. As mentioned before, it's just sucrose (white sugar) and high-fructose corn syrup (no relation to fruit fructose) that are the major villains to blood sugar control.

Grains are eliminated from many lean diets. I have kept whole grains, in small quantities in mine. Brown rice, whole wheat tortillas, and rye bread do not seem to raise my blood sugar, and the variety they provide would be hard for me to do without. This includes whole wheat pasta, although I eat far less than before, partly because without cheese, the appeal of many of these dishes is gone.

Included with the ground turkey we use as a ground beef substitute for un-grilled dishes, turkey bacon and chicken bratwurst have surprised me for their acceptability. We grill even these lean meats when possible. When it's not practical outside, we've found the George Foreman countertop grill to be fantastic.

The *organ meat* component of the *paleo* diet may be tough for me; but on the other hand, I'm eating many things I turned my nose up at before. I've watched the you-tube video a friend of mine shared on Facebook a couple of times. It's hard to stop thinking about it. "TEDxIowaCity - Dr. Terry Wahls - Minding Your Mitochondria" is the best snapshot of the science behind this kind of lean, hunter-gatherer paleo diet I've seen yet. It's also a great story. A western doctor who didn't accept the MS *sentence* she'd received, and found another way. MS, diabetes and a whole collection of chronic diseases are more related than we've traditionally thought. Diet shows up repeatedly as the key. The more cynical among us say these diet *cures* are ignored because they're not patentable. This one caught my attention because it's so close to what I've figured out for myself. Although I still eat more whole grains than Dr. Wahls recommends, and I'd need to nearly double my intake of vegetables, which is already much higher than my life before. Kale will be a challenge too; but, we just experimented with collard greens last night, cooked up with onion, quinoa, tomatoes, red chili, and some sliced up spicy chicken brats.

I can't deny that my relationship with food has substantially changed. Food is more in the *fuel for the body* category than the sensual experience it was most of my life. The foods with sugar and fat that I've given up are the ones that provide what I call *tastegasms*. It just comes for the first bite or two really (although we still eat the rest). There is plenty of enjoyment in the wonderful fruit and myriad great dishes that healthy food offers. But not that *over the top* sensation we get from the nasty stuff. I guess it all makes sense in the context of the addiction to fat and sugar that studies now prove is so common. Sex, gambling, drugs, or chocolate all amount to a roller coaster running from needful dip to eyes-rolled-back high. If you follow my path, you're going to level it all out. Steady as she goes. No hangovers or tastegasms, sustainable and good feeling.

~~~

Don't Settle For Spaghetti Sauce!
Beautiful, slightly wrinkled jalapenos, habaneros and roma tomatoes are in the perfect state for making salsa. They have ripened in the colander on the counter for several days. Any longer and some will go bad. But right now, the sweetness and flavor is at the max.
Fresh salsa is a joy and prime sustenance for Kathy and me. I started making it every week in 1997 when we moved to Colorado from Santa Fe and found that what everyone else called salsa here tasted more like spaghetti sauce to us. We eat and use gallons of the stuff. Besides with chips, mix it with avocados for some great guacamole. Top eggs or any meat with it. It's one of my pre-diabetes pleasures that's top-rated healthy.
It's hard to get the perfect consistency without a Cuisnart. I've got an 11 cup unit and here's how I make a full batch:
-toss in a few cloves of garlic and chop
-when habaneros are not in season, and the jalapenos and romas are average size, I use equal numbers, usually about 15 each. When I can get 2-3 habaneros, I cut the number of jalapenos in half.
Cut the stems off. Toss in the habaneros and chop. Toss in the jalapenos and chop.
-slice romas in 1/8's and toss 'em in, filling it up. There'll be 3-5 remaining.

-add a tablespoon of coarse salt, squeeze a whole lime into it, and add a couple of tablespoons of balsamic vinegar.

- chop exactly the right duration to NOT leave huge chunks and NOT make soup, about 8 seconds.

-Slice the remaining tomatoes (or as many as you can fit) in 1/8 's or 1/16 's and fill it up.

-chop just a few seconds. The nice thing about the Cuisnart is that the whole thing will get spinning in a really nice vortex that yields the perfect texture with practice.

This stuff will keep for at least 2 weeks in the fridge. We don't know if it will keep longer because it's always eaten by then.

WHAT PILLS TO TAKE

Ideally, we'd eat enough Kale, fish, blueberries and other super foods and not need supplements... but I know I can't eat that much Kale. It appears that the absorption is better from the natural sources, but in my opinion, getting some in a supplement is better than nothing. My goals for the supplements are threefold. I want to maintain a high intake of antioxidants and anything else that helps control the damage from high blood sugar. I also want to make use of anything that has reasonable evidence for helping to moderate blood sugar levels. The third type of supplement I take includes anything that might tackle the root autoimmune problem.

Jane, my acupuncturist, has a great knowledge of nutrition and supplements, and has helped me decide whether a news story about a supplement is worth pursuing, and what dosage makes sense. Fabio, my physician, helps confirm any conflicts with anything else I'm taking. He didn't originally put much stock in these, but if there was no harm and I didn't mind spending my money, he was OK with it.

Vitamin D has been the trendy supplement in the news for some time now. There is some data that even the hard core evidence-based guys like Fabio consider slightly promising for it. This quote from a 2010 press release sums it up pretty well.

Vitamin D insufficiency is a risk factor for a number of diseases and thus, is a growing concern worldwide, as approximately one billion people may be vitamin D deficient. However, the biological basis for vitamin D deficiency predisposing to disease is poorly understood.

It causes no harm, is relatively inexpensive, and is one of the few things that are suggested to help with autoimmune disorders. You can request a test for this when you get you blood work for A1c, C-peptide, or whatever. Per Jane's instructions I take 2000 IU per day.

Zinc falls in the damage control category. I spotted "Preventing diabetes damage: Zinc's effects on a kinky, two-faced cohort" in June, 2011, and was intrigued by the specific mechanism for Zinc's prevention of amylin clumping on the beta cells. If you read closely, you'll note you need to be careful of the dose. The study suggests that too much zinc can have exactly the opposite effect.

> *But when there's too much zinc around, all the binding sites in the middle positions are occupied and zinc must attach to amylin at the second site, which counteracts the effect of the first site. This may explain why decreased levels of insulin---the backup security guard---inside islet cells of diabetics result in islet cell death.*

The recommended dose for me for zinc is 15mg of zinc per day. As with any of these, you'll have to check with your doctor or someone with nutrition expertise to confirm what makes sense for you.

GABA is a long shot. But when I saw the *Chemical produced in pancreas prevented and reversed diabetes in mice* title of a press release in June, 2011, I was excited. It's already in vitamin stores, but for purposes of *calming*. But, once again, it's cheap, and Fabio and Jane could see no harm in adding it to my daily *gagathon*. Any of these that might stop the autoimmune attack AND regenerate the beta cells is a big deal.

> *The significance of GABA is that it corrects both known causes of Type 1 diabetes in mice: It works in the pancreas to regenerate insulin-producing beta cells and it acts on the immune system to*

stop the destruction of those cells. Those two actions are necessary to reverse the disease and prevent its recurrence. Until now, there has been no effective treatment that achieves both goals at the same time.

I may never know for sure, but GABA could actually be the one that reversed the damage to my pancreas. My GABA dosage is 1500mg per day.

N-A-C (N-acetyl-L-cysteine) is another supplement with a lot of conflicting buzz around it. It is reported to have both antioxidant and anti- inflammatory properties which benefit the immune system and is what caught my eye. It would fall mostly in the damage control category though, as per "Comparative Trial of N-Acetyl-Cysteine, Taurine, and Oxerutin on Skin and Kidney Damage in Long-Term Experimental Diabetes".

The findings that emerged from our study support the hypothesis that glomerular damage in diabetes can be prevented or at least attenuated by supplementation with specific antioxidants.

Some reports caution its use in conjunction with insulin. It's definitely another one to do some homework on. I currently take one 685mg capsule per day.

ALA (alpha-lipoic acid) appears to help in more than one way for diabetics. It's an antioxidant in the damage control group, but it also aids in blood sugar control according to "Substance used to treat complications from diabetes also proves to work as antioxidant."

Besides preventing neuropathy, alpha-lipoic acid is especially important for diabetics because it may improve blood-glucose control by improving insulin action while also inhibiting the oxidation of LDL cholesterol, which contributes to heart disease.

Diabetics are at increased risk of heart disease and have increased oxidative stress.

Jane's research on this one showed that I need to take 1200mg per day. It's only recently I found an economical 600mg tablet at the local health food store. Previously, only much lower doses were mass produced, leaving the choice between 6 pills a day or spending double for the boutique brand.

Fish Oil (Omega-3 EPA/DHA) seems to deserve all the praise it gets. "The secret to fish oil's anti-inflammatory properties" is an example of many studies that show its anti-inflammatory prowess and positive effect on insulin sensitivity.

Omega-3s are very potent activators of GPR120 on macrophages -- more potent than any other anti-inflammatory we've ever seen, said Jerrold Olefsky of the University of California, San Diego.

Some people say that the liquid form is absorbed more efficiently, but I just take three 1000mg softgels per day.

Vitamin B (Balanced B Complex) has no shocking or amazing promise for diabetics, although the biotin it contains is specifically linked with the production and release of insulin. When we're eating all the healthy, non-processed foods we should, we get all the vitamins we need. For me, this one is just a bit of a backup against any deficiencies. I buy a good quality tablet mostly because they don't stink, and I take one per day.

I've seen claims for other supplements like chromium, but at this point, I feel that since one or more of what I'm already taking is obviously working, why add anything? And besides, 12 pills a day are plenty. I'm better at it than I used to be but swallowing some of these is a pain. For some reason the light, clear capsules that my GABA and NAC come in are the worst. At least I don't spew it out any more when I gag. I clamp my hand over my mouth and force a massive swallow muscle flex to jam the little boogers down.

Since this section is technically titled "What Pills I Take", I'll mention the oral diabetes medications that I either took or still take. This can't be an advice section either because there are so many ways you may have gotten to where you are now, and only a good doctor can properly prescribe this stuff. Most Type 2's, mis-diagnosed LADA's, or insulin refusers like me start out on one or more of the common diabetes meds like metformin. It's proven, has data for good outcomes, and is cheap. Some people have stomach issues with it and have to find a substitute, but it's what I was prescribed, along with glipizide, at diagnosis in May, 2009. They work in various ways on the pancreas and liver and you can check out an authority like "pubmed.com" for all the details if you want. A Type 2 might be on something like metformin forever if they make moderate changes to their lifestyle. They might be able to quit it if they radically fix their diet and cure themselves (best option). The worst outcome for a Type 2 would mean be to make no lifestyle changes and get to quit metformin, but only because they have to start shooting insulin. A normal Type 1 won't ever take the pills because the theory is there's no pancreas function left for the metformin (or whatever) to stimulate. The oddball LADA's like me, if they don't start insulin immediately, take the pills for a year or two until they don't help any more, and then go to insulin. My path was exactly like that EXCEPT that when the metformin and glipizide became less effective, I researched and began doing everything I'm detailing in this book. Last summer (2011), when my A1c dropped into the normal range, I quit the glipizide. Amazingly, my numbers were not affected. In December 2011, I cut the metformin by 25% down to 1500 mg per day. After 2 months, and blood sugar still well controlled, I cut it another 25%, down to 1000mg per day. By the time you're reading this, hopefully I'll be off it altogether. This success with discontinuing the diabetes oral medications is more of the reason why I believe my pancreas is alive and recovering. Fabio, my physician, has been aware, and comfortable with each decrease in my medications.

There's my list. I suppose some new study about something otherwise harmless that is shown to help with my goals of damage control, BS control, and autoimmune system help might be enough for me to add something. But I'd rather cut down if I can figure out which things are actually working. Theoretically, if my BS stays controlled indefinitely, the damage control (antioxidants) wouldn't be needed. On the other hand, most of this stuff is touted for other benefits in addition to those that are diabetes specific.

WHAT ELSE TO DO EVERY DAY

After diet and supplements, the other two critica
supports to this 4-legged stool we're going to set our
healthy butt on are *activity* and *stress reduction*. As I said i
introduction, libraries are full of and more will be writte
about stress reduction. It's by far the area that will require
the most customization to find your solution. But
remember, this book is like Captain Barbosa's description
of the Pirate Code, "It's more of a guideline" than a
specific set of rules.

I use the word *activity* instead of *exercise* because the
evidence (published and my own) shows that as far as
controlling blood sugar and maintaining a balanced
metabolism goes, you don't have to have hours of an
aerobic, sweat-soaked workout. If you're trying to lose
weight in addition to managing your diabetes, than you will
have to get breathless regularly. But not for glycemic
control. Many people end up doing less because they think
they have to make such a big production out of it. They
don't have time to go for a run, or the weather is bad, so
they don't do anything. I hate to run, or do many of the
classic workout activities. Instead, I try to be active in little
ways throughout the day. I run up and down the stairs
every single time, all day long. I walk each garbage can to
the end of the drive instead of using the car. I use a walk-
behind mower instead of a riding tractor most of the time. I
play golf on the Wii and jog in place in between shots.

A couple of formal 20 minute (minimum) activities in
addition to the *all the time* stair type stuff will round out your
plan. I do 30 minutes of a combination Wii yoga/strength
workout almost every day (occasionally miss a Saturday or
Sunday). A 20 minute speed walk is perfect when weather
permits. I actually go out and throw horse shoes by myself
for 30 minutes as fast as I can and get a little upper body

ᵃ. Just be creative and look for all
ᵉnt themselves throughout most

ᴛenth time that finding a way to
dark horse in this game. I knew I
ᵣ before all this, but I thought I handled
ᵢ surprised at the improvement in my
physical health that seems directly attributable
ᵍ some major changes in how I react to *life*. There
ᵗle bit of the *which came first, chicken or egg* question
ᵉre. Jane has this simple, elegant theory about "angry",
inflamed cells affecting our conscious reactions at least as
much as being an angry and stressed out person affects our
immune system and organ function. It makes a lot of sense.
There's every indication that both aspects are equally
interconnected. It's certainly in line with what I've gleaned
so far about Eastern medicine. But philosophical questions
aside, it's clear that we have to tackle the physical and
mental aspects simultaneously.

The easier, daily things you can do to de-stress include
yoga and meditation. I usually use the term yoga to refer to
the exercises, or *asana*, part of yoga science. Yoga exercises
are a lot of bang for the buck because they fulfill both the
activity and de-stress needs of this plan. Many activities are
stress relievers, but the breath, balance, and mind calming
of asana can't be beat. I also took another piece of advice
from Swamiji, my guru friend, and added a *prana* exercise to
my daily regimen. Prana are the specific breath control
exercises that comprise another whole area of the science
of yoga. I actually incorporate the idea of breath control
into my entire day and everything I do. After a few months,
it has become somewhat automatic to moderate, equalize,
and use my breath for more than respiration. The theory
behind prana is that while we have very little conscious
control over many bodily functions like heart rate and

digestion, we can exercise control over our breathing. Breath becomes the interface between the physical and the *qi* (pronounced chee) energy. Any control we gain over balancing qi gives us a tool for balancing the rest of our body and mind functions. It's not my goal here to create yoga devotees, it just seems to work for me. Check it out if you want. For me, both the asana and prana are useful as pragmatic, defined, *do it no matter what's happening with the day* habits that are easier to remember than some of the other attitude adjustments I've undertaken.

Don't skip this section! Even though it's about meditation, and you don't care about any of that *foo foo* stuff right? You just want the diet, the supplements, the concrete, actionable things that make some sense to our western mindsets. Well here's the deal. Others have done close enough variations of this diet and supplements and not succeeded in the long term goals. Particularly, when it comes to fending off and reversing the autoimmune attack, there's not a doubt in my mind that stress is a predominant driver and that acupuncture, yoga, and meditation are unmatched in their ability to moderate it. I also do not write off the possibility that these practices act in more direct ways to re-balance physical processes. I think the fact that eastern medicine looks at entire organ systems as a unit versus the narrow target of any western pharmacology makes perfect sense when considering something like the pancreas. It has a complex integration with the rest of the organs in the gut as well as the brain. After reading some of the science, I get the impression that the state of knowledge around insulin secretion and receptivity is like it is for physics. A lot of discrete functions are explored, but I haven't seen an entire process map yet.

In any case, whatever western medicine knows, there's still no cure for autoimmune diabetes. There will be one at some point, but I know it'll cost more than 15 minutes of meditation a day. As long as we're talking cost, know that good acupuncture will cost you $60 an hour. If you do it weekly as I did for the first 10 months of my plan, it qualifies as a significant investment. It's a leap of faith. It's not like a western pill that will actively make you feel something (good or bad) in a short enough time to register with our western attention spans. You *will* probably feel great after each session, but the real action is happening in an entirely *other* body realm. I cut back to every 2-3 weeks a couple of months ago for purely financial reasons, and I regret it. Every time now that my blood sugar is up a little I wonder just how much of a sustaining force the acupuncture is. And to what extent will curtailing of it unbalance this miracle of the resurgence of my supposedly dead pancreas.

~~~

I have created a force field
It resides within, and acts upon my body
all the parts to build it were already in there, but
they were an awful mess
toxic crud scraping is long, hard work
at first the light was bad, A/C was broken
an acupuncturist had to rebuild the wiring harness
while I went in search of the power source
rumor had it that we all had one
a universal port
so I started rummaging around
and there it was, in the far corner
under loads of dirty laundry
and so dim as to appear unremarkable
but once shoveled, swept, scrubbed and polished
a pure beam emanated
infusing the entire space and powering up

my force field contraption
which proceeds to marinate my kidneys
liver, spleen, and recalcitrant pancreas
in a bath of anti-waywardness
re-establishing a flow here
moderating a torrent there
easing pressure on worn hinges
clearing filters, the list goes on

I just worry a little
at the rube Goldberg nature of the device
I don't REALLY know exactly how it works
I know it's pretty damn picky about what I eat
and it's ultra-sensitive to the un-cool
especially those self-destructive things
that we love to do, think the keywords
anger, pain, and victim

but the thing runs, the force field holds
keeping my 20th century guts running like clockwork
I guess I'll just cross my fingers
and keep pouring in what's lean, green and chill
exercising and meditating daily
even when the pot's boiling over
claiming to be more immediate

~~~

The meditation piece is interesting. I originally didn't hold out much hope that it would help. The part of the brain controlling any of the feedback and regulation connected with metabolism and/or the pancreas seemed too far below the conscious level to be actionable. I now know there are several flaws in that assumption, but what made me change my mind about trying was the story of

Wim Hof, "The Iceman". Hof was known before this for his feats of enduring cold. He can be covered in ice cubes for 90 minutes, run a marathon above the arctic circle barefoot and in only shorts, and more. He taught himself *tummo*, a Tibetan meditation technique that gives him control over body functions that this new study showed includes immune response. The study, "Research On 'Iceman' Wim Hof Suggests It May Be Possible to Influence Autonomic Nervous System and Immune Response", using an immune-response producing endotoxin, certainly looks legitimate. Hof was able to lower his body's immune response by 50% compared to 240 other subjects by using concentration and meditation. Even though Hof mastered this technique on his own, the normal path is through 12 years in a monastery in the Himalayas. I have no presumption that I will ever actually achieve real tummo control. But my research has found studies showing that even plain old mindfulness meditation has health benefits, including significant stress reduction. This one's really kind of a no-brainer. The price is right. And if you really look at your day, there's 15 minutes there somewhere. Most people could cut back their Facebook time by that much and be no worse for it.

You can find plenty of books and googled information on meditation techniques. You can pay for or find a free class. You can get candles and incense and symbolic art to stare at to help you focus. Whatever works. I just sit in a chair in a quiet place, eyes closed. I relax my muscles one side at a time. I focus on breath, keeping inhale and exhale even. I think about the breath pulling in energy that flows up my spine, washing across all my organs with a cleansing light. The exhale takes away any impurities. When my mind wanders to the mundane, daily stuff, as it constantly does, I acknowledge the thought and return focus to breath. It's easier some days than others.

You have to figure out how to do these things every day. Finding a sustainable healthy lifestyle means making some choices you can live with indefinitely. You might have to change a job, or a relationship. I hope not. But what's more important than your health and happiness?

Agenda For a Healthy Day – Winter Version

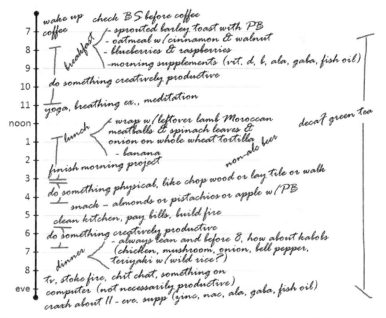

Here's an example of putting it all together. How to live a day that's part of a sustainable life. It details the lean diet, regular activity, and low-stress environment that have brought my mind and body to the best state ever. Something about this routine even reversed an autoimmune disease. But don't wait for that excuse. This isn't that extreme. It's my recipe, you'll have to tweak it for yourself. If you can't work from home, for example, you'll have to figure out how to fit it all. As long as your work isn't a stressor. If it is, you'll have to fix that too.

WILL YOU LIKE THE NEW YOU

Nobody's going to argue with the strength, balance, reduced illness, and Zen cool attitude that results from doing all this. But is it worth it? Will you still be You?

I won't lie. You will not be exactly the same person when you arrive at your destination. Is the amazing physical and mental health a tradeoff for part of your soul? Obviously, you know my answer to these questions or I wouldn't be suggesting this road is worth travelling. So the question is what kinds of things are different and why won't you miss them?

I was talking to my mom on the phone the other day and at one point she said, "You know one thing that's different about you? You wait for me to respond now." She'd spotted a difference in me. I know I'm calmer and less prone to anger, but I hadn't thought about how this new *patience* affects every interaction I have. For me, calmer equals being a little kinder, and that must translate into being a better listener. Now Kathy (my wife) might read this and laugh her ass off, saying "You've got a ways to go." And she's right. Actually, if you ask Kathy about how I've changed, she'll say it's a mixed bag. She's glad to have me healthy and likes the more even temperament. But on some days (that are hopefully growing fewer) she'll admit to missing the *old* Russell. When pressed, she'll bemoan the apparent *all about Russell* nature of much of this last year. While every relationship will handle this differently, the challenge of tearing down and rebuilding yourself and NOT being self-absorbed while doing it will be faced by all. In my case, I was self-centered to begin with. Combining that with the decision to try to record, communicate and advocate my findings means I really have my work cut out for me.

I'm heartened though by my family's comparisons to normalcy. I know that the other road, the one originally paved with insulin would've brought us to a very different place. Talk about life revolving around me! With vials in the fridge and syringe or pumps and meters constantly present, there would be no level playing field comparisons to the life before. The transition to this clean lifestyle has not been as jolting as the usual diabetic resignation to a sentence of house arrest as a chronic disease victim. Remember I said I'd be bad-mouthing your inner victim pretty regularly? That guy can cripple you at virtually every turn.

So have I answered the question "Will you like the new you?"

If you say I have, go back and read this section again. I can't possibly answer that question for you. Just like the rest of the information in this book, my experience can only provide hints, a rough treasure map that a crazy sailor you don't know from Adam has given you. Even if you find the pieces of eight, will they bring you happiness? Obviously, I think they will. I wouldn't bother to spill my guts to the rabble otherwise.

HOW LONG IS FOREVER

Journey, path, road, plan, and experiment are all terms I've used to describe how I've changed my life. I need to be clear that there is no destination or end point that will mean it's all over and you can *relax*. You're going to be on the road the rest of your life. I'm talking about devising a mode of travel that's relaxing en route. I overuse the word sustainable. But all the pearls of wisdom we hear about living in the moment, and for today, are right. Live now. Find a way to be happy now.

~~~

The Gift of Diabetes

I asked the universe, unknowingly
to give me a tool to help change my life
something to remind me, daily
to rock steady and stride beyond temptation
I asked for immediate feedback
to the ultimate question
"Have I cared for my body/mind so righteously well today
that I deserve great health?"

~~~

I'm not saying you won't continue to make adjustments for years. As your body learns to trust you, it might cut you a little slack. Just exercise extreme caution in any compromises to your initial plan. If you've managed to stabilize your blood sugar and your pancreas is mostly doing its job, you've already used your one *Get Out of Jail Free* card. Assume you won't get a second chance. If your body offers up a helpful change, humbly accept it and don't abuse it. After about 8 months on my plan, I noticed my body was a little more forgiving about between meal snacks. I could go from breakfast to lunch more often without needing a midmorning snack to keep from feeling low. At the beginning, if I were going to out on errands for a few hours, I had to take some fruit and nuts with me. Now, if I forget, I don't have to turn around and go get it. I've already mentioned the *Champagne Exception* I eventually worked into my alcohol ban. Just be careful. Is a little compromise going to escalate? Here's my rationale on these experimental adjustments. First of all, nothing like this should be tried until all pangs and cravings are long gone. I'm not sure I'd ever experiment with sugar. It's too poisonous. Fudge is too insidious. I would want to eat it just because of it. Not like the champagne. I don't crave alcohol anymore. The reason I've chosen to occasionally drink it is because of its social value. I would never drink it alone. I can't say the same thing about fudge.

If you have Diabetes, you are lucky. It gives us a concrete reason for being the happiest smurfs on the block, because a positive attitude is directly and measurably linked to keeping us healthy. The stress of all non-optimistic directions will set off our blood sugar alarms. This instant feedback is a hell of a compass. I know I wouldn't have made the right choices for living without this gun at the back of my head.

If you still roll your eyes at that sort of drivel, that's OK. It just means you haven't completely closed the door in the face of your victim yet. As long as he thinks you've got a waver left in you, he'll come knocking. Days your blood sugar is over 200, or when the girl scout cookies arrive or there's a new microbrew at the local pub are all opportunities to spot any dry rot in your foundation. Just like any repair, it's the prep work that can make or break the job. It's tempting to just spackle around some of the seemingly bedrock pieces of who you are. They seem immovable. Alcohol and full fat foods were part of my persona. I've had to change or delete many of the truisms and opinions I had before. I was proud of my knowledge of rum and beer, and my ability to quaff mass quantities in a manly American manner. I scoffed at low-fat anything, foregoing ice cream if it wasn't full butter fat.

An early blog post of mine was titled, Burning My Superman Card. It gets at this idea of giving up things that had appeared to be part of the root definition of myself. In my case, before Diabetes, I believed I was a bit of a superman. I never broke a bone, have few cavities, rarely got sick, ate anything I wanted without weight gain or other effect (I thought). I believed I was positioned to be the ultimate survivor. I wasn't dependent on any medications, was a camel, could go all day without food if necessary. That was a large part of who I thought I was, that sense of invulnerability. And I've had to cut that piece of me out and toss it.

Discovering I was mortal saved me. It has calmed my ego and moderated the self-centeredness that allowed a kinder me to evolve. A kinder me was key to reducing stress. Less stress has been critical in reversing my LADA. A less stressful me is also better for my family and the rest of the universe.

The pieces of me that I've tossed out have turned out to be the less honest bits anyway. They were not really life-supporting. They weren't really sustainable. They used more energy than they conserved. I'm travelling light now. Everything in the trunk has to contribute. I can't afford to haul around any half-assed convictions. If you want, think of it this way. You're rebuilding your jalopy for the road trip to forever. You pull it apart, clean up the corroded parts, put it all back together and parts are left over. What to do? Just toss 'em.

So how long is forever?

If you've rebuilt your ride without shortcuts, are adding clean fuel, have the top down, and are laughing along with the right companions, it's not long enough.

REFERENCES

Autoimmune disorders,
http://www.nlm.nih.gov/medlineplus/ency/article/000816.htm

Dutch professor: Type 1 diabetes can be cured,
http://www.rnw.nl/africa/node/621976

Study finds some insulin production in long-term Type 1 diabetes,
http://www.eurekalert.org/pub_releases/2012-02/mgh-sfs021512.php

"TEDxIowaCity - Dr. Terry Wahls - Minding Your Mitochondria,
http://www.youtube.com/watch?v=KLjgBLwH3Wc&list=HL1323189656&feature=mh_lolz

Vitamin D linked to autoimmune and cancer disease genes, underscoring risks of deficiency,
http://www.eurekalert.org/pub_releases/2010-08/cshl-vdl081710.php

Preventing diabetes damage: Zinc's effects on a kinky, two-faced cohort,
http://www.eurekalert.org/pub_releases/2011-06/uom-pdd063011.php

Chemical produced in pancreas prevented and reversed diabetes in mice,
http://www.eurekalert.org/pub_releases/2011-06/smh-cpi062811.php

Comparative Trial of N-Acetyl-Cysteine, Taurine, and Oxerutin on Skin and Kidney Damage in Long-Term Experimental Diabetes,
http://diabetes.diabetesjournals.org/content/52/2/499

Substance used to treat complications from diabetes also proves to work as antioxidant,
http://www.eurekalert.org/pub_releases/1999-11/UoTS-Sutt-111199.php

The secret to fish oil's anti-inflammatory properties,
http://www.eurekalert.org/pub_releases/2010-09/cp-tst083010.php

Research On 'Iceman' Wim Hof Suggests It May Be Possible to Influence Autonomic Nervous System and Immune Response,
http://www.sciencedaily.com/releases/2011/04/110422090203.htm?utm_source=feedburner&utm_medium=feed&utm_campaign=Feed%3A+sciencedaily+%28ScienceDaily%3A+Latest+Science+News%29

###

About Russell Stamets

Before the universe assigned him the Diabetes project, Russell spent a fairly geeky 20 years in training and healthcare. His move to full-time writing in November 2011 was facilitated by a layoff after 10 years as Education Director at a community hospital. He also gained firsthand experience with the previous recession in 2002, when he closed his Boulder, CO based computer training business. If he was crazy enough to list on a resume other stretches of his odd path, it would include office manager, bookkeeper, taxi driver, framer, plasterer, ski instructor, and bugler at Santa Fe Downs.

Russell is currently taking his own advice, pivoting away from his high stress corporate and management experience. With their youngest off to college next fall, Russell and wife Kathy are selling the house, and proceeding with their plan to purchase and move aboard an east coast based sailboat.

Russell welcomes your correspondence and can be reached several ways, including:
Blog: russellstamets.blogspot.com
Email: russell.stamets@gmail.com
Twitter: @russellstamets
Facebook: www.facebook.com/russellkstamets
LinkedIn: www.linkedin.com/in/russellkstamets

Printed in Great Britain
by Amazon